I0711059

DEPRESSION
A SIMPLE WAY OUT

Simple steps for overcoming depressive disorder

Bright Benny

All rights reserved 2024
Bright Benny

TABLE CONTENTS

Presentation

Depression can be a crippling and difficult disease that can fundamentally influence our connections and capacity to work. While trouble might be one of the trademark qualities of sadness, there is likewise a star grouping of negative mind-sets, unforgiving reasoning examples and lessened inspiration. The individual frequently feels powerless, discouraged,and crushed, which prompts withdrawal from life exercises. Side effects could become serious and lead to death or self destruction.

The beginning of depression happens when excruciating topics are set off. One subject includes a feeling of disappointment in life errands, joined by insecurities. The other significant subject in despondency is misfortune. This is joined by recollections of past misfortune and profound sensations of weakness.

After an intensive evaluation of side effects and pain points, we attempt to accomplish fast side effect, help by utilizing mental and experiential systems, which will assist clients with growing more adaptable and humane convictions to liberate them from depression.

CHAPTER ONE

Depression: Overview

Depressive disorder is a typical mental problem. It includes a discouraged state of mind or loss of delight or interest in exercises for significant stretches of time. Depression is not the same as standard temperament changes and sentiments about daily existence. It can influence all parts of life, incorporating associations with family, companions and local area. It can result from or lead to issues at school and at work.

Depression can happen to anybody. Individuals who have survived misuse, extreme misfortunes or other upsetting occasions are bound to foster wretchedness. Ladies are bound to have discouragement than men.

Roughly 280 million individuals on the planet have melancholy (1). Despondency is around half more normal among ladies than among men. Around the world, over 10% of pregnant ladies and ladies who have quite recently conceived an offspring experience melancholy (2). In excess of 700 000 individuals bite the dust because of self destruction consistently. Self destruction is the fourth driving reason for death in 15-29-year-olds.

Despite the fact that there are known, compelling medicines for mental problems, over 75% of individuals in low-and center pay nations get no treatment (3). Obstructions to successful consideration remember an absence of speculation for emotional well-being care, absence of prepared medical services suppliers and social disgrace related with mental problems.

CHAPTER TWO

Causes of Depression

Depression might actually be brought about by the accompanying:

Pregnancy and conceiving an offspring

A few ladies are especially powerless against depressive disorder after pregnancy. The hormonal and actual changes, as well as the additional obligation of another life, can prompt post pregnancy anxiety. In some cases depression begins before you conceive an offspring. Depression in pregnancy is known as antenatal gloom.

Menopause

Menopause is the point at which your periods stop because of lower chemical levels. At times menopause can set off gloom, especially in the initial not many years.

Menopause can likewise cause side effects, for example, trouble and emotional episodes. Emotional wellness side effects brought about by menopause are unique in relation to wretchedness.

Forlornness

Feeling forlorn, brought about by things, for example, becoming cut off from your loved ones, can build your gamble of sadness.

Liquor and medications

At the point when life is getting them down, certain individuals attempt to adapt by drinking a lot of liquor or ingesting medications. This can bring about a winding of melancholy.

Marijuana can assist you with unwinding, however there's proof that it can likewise welcome on sadness, especially in teens.

"Suffocating your distresses" with a beverage is likewise not suggested. Liquor influences the science of the cerebrum, which builds the gamble of gloom.

Sickness

You might have a higher gamble of misery assuming you have a longstanding or hazardous sickness, for example, coronary illness, malignant growth or a condition that causes long haul torment.

Head wounds are likewise a frequently under-perceived reason for sorrow. A serious head injury can set off temperament swings and profound issues.

In certain individuals an underactive thyroid (hypothyroidism) can cause misery.

CHAPTER THREE

Social Media Influence

Today is no secret that the society is innovatively progressed and that worldwide everybody has a cell phone or other handheld electronic devices. Individuals can now have many choices readily available in no time flat. Albeit the innovation is useful, overabundance use of virtual entertainment, like Facebook, Twitter, WhatsApp, and so forth, can be identical to enslavement and adversely influences individuals. Strikingly, numerous people who invest the vast majority of their energy on these applications have been found to have nervousness and depression related side effects. Subsequently, obviously the expanded utilization of web-based entertainment in contemporary society unfavorably influences people bringing about despondency and uneasiness, especially in the people who use it for a lengthy period consistently.

The dislodging speculation asserts that unreasonable contribution in certain exercises deters support in different exercises that might be more useful. Albeit this hypothesis originates before virtual entertainment, it can assist with making sense of why inordinate social media entertainment utilization may be hurtful. As per the thought, consistently invested social media removes energy required for exercises that are better for an individual's psychological well-being, like activity. This suggests that the mischief delivered by virtual entertainment is relative to how much time spent on it, reinforcing the case that "social media entertainment is unsafe to a person's emotional wellness". This affirms the relocation speculation's depiction of how virtual entertainment uproots positive exercises, having a negative, monotonic effect on emotional well-being, demonstrating and affirming the statement that web-based entertainment causes sadness and nervousness.

Extreme utilization of web-based entertainment can hurt a singular's insight and feeling of confinement. Also, people are passing up time that they could be spending on different exercises, including considering, dozing, investing quality energy with loved ones, partaking in sports, or essentially resting. Puberty is famous for remaining up much past their regular sleep time, bringing about an absence of legitimate rest reliably today. They are persistently immersing their cerebrums with data that should be arranged and handled. It is all around acknowledged that rest is essential for the body and the cerebrum to perform at their best. Lack of sleep has additionally been connected with higher frequencies of depression before. Moreover, lower scholastic execution depression is straightforwardly connected with how much time an understudy spends via social media entertainment stages like Facebook and Twitter.

One more quality of virtual entertainment use is that it altogether affects mental self portrait and self-esteem, which are vigorously impacted by self-perception. The picture of the body alludes to how an individual perspectives oneself overall and what they hold to be true with regards to it, including actual characteristics and mentalities toward it. Many individuals are engrossed with their actual engaging quality and disregard their intrinsic abilities to acquire cultural acknowledgment. More often than not, regardless of whether they get recognition or measure up to society's assumptions, it isn't sufficient, so they set out on a mission to be pretty much as wonderful as a model or entertainer, which prompts despondency. Via online entertainment stages like Snapchat, Instagram, Pinterest, and Tumblr, various male and female models' bodies are shown. Thus, in the event that individuals neglect to match online entertainment's assumptions, nervousness concerns might happen, prompting wretchedness.

Moreover, depression and nervousness can oppress anybody, paying little heed to progress in years, religion, or social standing. These days, a big part of the superstars experience the ill effects of misery and nervousness, very much like every other person. Individuals are interminably bewildered by the distinction among distress and despondency; they accept that a discouraged individual seems miserable, however this isn't true. Additionally, celebrities seem, by all accounts, to be happy before the camera and the media, yet they are experiencing within, which is obscure to the general population. Indeed, even large numbers of them have ended it all because of discouragement, which was exacerbated to some degree by the utilization of online entertainment stages. Furthermore, due to the present online entertainment situated culture, they may likewise get messages from their naysayers who might be discourteous to them or do something hurtful to their standing. Therefore, celebrities who get negative remarks via online entertainment are regularly compelled to have some time off from their professions, prompting wretchedness.

Taking everything into account, the over the top virtual entertainment use can unfavorably affect people. Its constant openness to clients can exasperate the nervousness and despondency related side effects. Moreover, it is expressed that the impacts of virtual entertainment use by people are subject to whether they use it helpfully or unfavorably. Generally, depressiion and nervousness are portrayed by diminished correspondence with individuals, investing more energy alone at home, and having awful considerations. A discouraged individual's dear companion or relative can help them in escaping their psychological problems by empowering or spurring them to productively utilize online entertainment. The posts and stories via virtual entertainment can altogether affect one's sensations of gloom and uneasiness. Accordingly, individuals should perceive the need of limiting their utilization of web-based entertainment and taking part in actual work to make their psyches less focused and better

CHAPTER FOUR

Symptoms of Depression

Depression is a complex psychological wellness condition that makes an individual have a low state of mind and may leave them feeling constantly miserable or sad.

Symptoms can be a transitory involvement with reaction to sadness or injury. Be that as it may, in the event that they last longer than about fourteen days, they might show a serious burdensome issue.

These side effects can likewise show other emotional well-being conditions, for example, bipolar turmoil and post-horrible pressure issue.

A portion of the side effects of despondency of wretchedness: discouraged temperament as a general rule, including sensations of pity or vacancy loss of delight in already charming exercises excessively little or a lot of rest most days accidental weight reduction or gain or changes in hunger actual fomentation or sensations of drowsiness low energy or weakness sensations of uselessness or responsibility inconvenience focusing or simply deciding nosy contemplations of death or self destruction.

The symptoms fluctuate among people and may change over the long haul. For a specialist to analyze wretchedness, an individual priority at least five side effects that are available during a similar 2-week time span.

Different side effects are likewise present, which might include:

- unfortunate focus
- sensations of extreme culpability or low self-esteem
- sadness about what's to come
- considerations about kicking the bucket or self destruction
- disturbed rest
- changes in craving or weight
- feeling extremely drained or low in energy.
- Misery can cause challenges in all parts of life, remembering for the local area and at home, work and school.

Depression can be classified as gentle, moderate, or extreme relying upon the number and seriousness of side effects, as well as the effect on the singular's working.
There are various examples of depressiion including:

1. single episode depression, meaning the individual's solitary episode;
2. repetitive depression problem, meaning the individual has a background marked by no less than two depression episodes; and
3. bipolar turmoil, implying that depression episodes
4. substitute with times of hyper side effects, which incorporate elation or crabbiness, expanded 5 or energy, and different side effects like expanded chattiness, hustling contemplations, expanded confidence, diminished need for rest, distractibility, and hasty wild way of behaving.

CHAPTER FIVE

The Connection between Physical and Psychological Wellness

It is critical to note that remaining healthy is a necessary part of many people's lives. The need for wellbeing guidance is clear all over; be that as it may, the vast majority of this data centers around the body. Physical and psychological wellness are firmly related. People will endure assuming that their physical or psychological well-being is noticeably off.

There, right off the bat, is a positive relationship among depression and a singular's insusceptible framework.

The ailment impacts one's inspiration and state of mind as well as can overpower Lymphocyte reactions to microscopic organisms and infections, an issue that could cause one to stay wiped out for longer. A person with a powerless framework could likewise acquire different diseases, like asthma or sensitivities. A few scientists have likewise placed that the resistant reaction could bring about misery. In such an occasion, a provocative response might prompt discouragement.

Moreover, weariness and psychological instability might introduce inferable from uneasiness, sorrow, and mind-set problems. An individual would feel depleted and tired based of these issues. Moreover, nervousness, outrage, and heart wellbeing are connected with psychological well-being. Nervousness, stress, and unexpected eruptions of fury might bring about heart issues, for example, coronary failures. It is vital to bring down nervousness levels to lighten sensations of weakness in spite of being quietly associated.

The association among discouragement and actual Issues
despondency is ordinarily connected with different side effects, like culpability, pity, sadness, and peevishness. Other normal side effects of gloom incorporate focusing on undertakings or inconvenience centering. Melancholy could likewise bring about stomach issues, agony, anxiety, and weakness. It is likewise fundamental to consider the potential for melancholy medicines as such

drug might have actual incidental effects, for example, sexual brokenness, weight change, and queasiness.

An individual might encounter torment, displaying agonies and throbs that influence their appendages, back, or joints. A few people foster weakening and constant body torment, which might prompt melancholy, however the reason and impacts might be opposite in nature. A few people accept that depression brings about individuals encountering torment diversely as an individual might have a lower torment resistance and low agony limit when contrasted with their countrymen that are not discouraged. Depression is additionally connected with different issues, like lower back torment and persistent irritation.

It is additionally fundamental to consider that people with depressiion have predictable gastrointestinal side effects, for example, swelling, sickness, blockage, or looseness of the bowels. One potential explanation such issues create is because of a synapse in the mind known as serotonin. This cerebrum synthetic is associated with melancholy as supporting controlling mood is accepted. Serotonin likewise assumes a huge part in directing stomach related capability. It is regularly put away in the stomach and has different ramifications for despondency.

CHAPTER SIX

Ways of coping with Depression

You can do whatever it takes to adapt to and explore gloom. Little changes to your day to day daily schedule, diet, and way of life propensities can all emphatically influence you.

There are little advances you can take to assist you with acquiring organization in your life and work on your feeling of prosperity.

Peruse on to figure out how to consolidate these methodologies such that seems OK for you.

1. Meet yourself where you are.

Depression influences a great many individuals, which may include you or those close to you. You may not understand they face comparable difficulties, feelings, and snags. Being open, tolerating, and cherishing toward yourself and what you're going through may assist you with exploring wretchedness.

Consistently with this problem is unique. It's essential to view your emotional wellness in a serious way and acknowledge that where you are correct now isn't where you'll continuously be.

2. Consider a stroll around the block

On days when you believe you can't get up, exercise might seem like the last thing you'd need to do. Yet, practice and active work can assist with diminishing side effects of discouragement and further develop energy levels. That's what research proposes, for certain individuals, exercise can be essentially as successful as medicine at easing depression side effects.

In any event, when you feel you can't or have little energy, check whether you'd do something contrary to everything your state of mind says to you to do. All things being equal, put forth a little objective for yourself, like strolling around the block.

3. Realize that today isn't characteristic of tomorrow

Inside feelings and considerations can change from one day to another. Following encounters through journaling or keeping a state of mind journal can assist you with recollecting this.

Assuming you were fruitless at getting up or achieving objectives today, recall that you haven't lost the upcoming chance to attempt once more.

Give yourself the effortlessness to acknowledge that while certain days will be troublesome, others will likewise be less troublesome. Attempt to anticipate the upcoming new beginning.

4. Survey the parts as opposed to summing up the entirety

Misery can hint memories with troublesome feelings. You might end up zeroing in on things that are pointless or seen as troublesome.

Attempt to stop this overgeneralization. Drive yourself to perceive the upside. On the off chance that it helps, compose why was the occasion or day significant. You can follow what you accomplished that day and which exercises were agreeable.

Seeing the weight you're providing for one thing might assist you with coordinating your considerations from the entire and to the singular pieces that were useful.

5. Do something contrary to what the 'downturn voice' recommends

The programmed, on accommodating voice in your mind might work you out of self improvement. Yet, assuming you figure out how to perceive this voice, you can figure out how to deal with it.

On the off chance that you accept an occasion won't be tomfoolery or worth your time, tell yourself, "You may be correct, yet it'll be preferable over staying here one more evening." You may before long see that programmed believed isn't useful all of the time.

6. Put forth achievable objectives

Rather than incorporating a not insignificant rundown of undertakings, think about putting forth little objectives that are more easily attainable. Putting forth and achieving these objectives can give a feeling of control and achievement and help with inspiration.

Feasible objectives might include:

- *Try not to clean the house; take the garbage out.*

- *Try not to do all the clothing that is stacked up; sort the heaps for some other time.*

- *Try not to get out your whole email inbox; simply address any time-delicate messages.*

At the point when you've done something insignificant, put your focus on another little thing, and afterward another. Along these lines, you have a rundown of unmistakable accomplishments and not an immaculate plan for the day.

7. Reward your endeavors

All objectives deserve acknowledgment, and all triumphs truly deserve festivity. At the point when you accomplish an objective, put forth a valiant effort to remember it. You may not want to celebrate with a cake and confetti, yet perceiving your own victories can be an incredible asset over any form negativity that accompanies depression. The memory of an incredible piece of handiwork might be particularly strong against pointless self-talk and overgeneralization.

8. Make an everyday practice

In the event that depression side effects disturb your everyday daily practice, a delicate timetable might assist you with feeling in charge. These plans don't need to outline a whole day.
Center around making a free however organized everyday practice to assist you with keeping your day to day pace.

9. Accomplish something you appreciate

Depression can push you to yield to your weariness. It might feel more remarkable than favored feelings.

Attempt to push back and accomplish something you love — something pleasurable or significant. It very well may be playing an instrument, painting, climbing, or trekking.

Participating in significant exercises lifts your state of mind or energy, which can additionally propel you to keep on taking part in exercises that assistance with exploring side effects.

10. Pay attention to music

Shows music can work on your state of mind and side effects of wretchedness. It might likewise reinforce your gathering of positive feelings.

Music can be particularly useful when acted in social environments, like a melodic group or band.

You can likewise receive a portion of similar benefits essentially by tuning in.

11. Invest energy in nature

Time in nature can impact an individual's state of mind. Research proposes that strolls in nature might work on burdensome side effects in individuals with clinical melancholy.

Time in regular spaces might further develop temperament and perception and lower the gamble of psychological wellness problems. In any case, there's just restricted research on the immediate impact of nature on those with clinical discouragement.

Think about going for a stroll at lunch among the trees or investing energy in your nearby park. Or on the other hand plan an end of the week climb. These exercises can help you reconnect with nature and absorb a few beams simultaneously.

12. Invest energy with friends and family

Depression can entice you to separate yourself and pull out from individuals you love and trust, however up close and personal time can assist with washing away those inclinations.

In the event that you can't hang out face to face, calls or video talks can likewise be useful.

Attempt to remind yourself these individuals care about you. Oppose the compulsion to feel like you're a weight. You want the cooperation — and they probably do as well.

13. Express your sentiments

Think about composition or journaling about the thing you're encountering. Then, when the sentiments lift, expound on that as well. Research proposes that keeping a diary can be a useful extra technique for overseeing emotional well-being conditions.

Recording your contemplations can assist you with communicating what you're feeling all the more obviously. It can likewise assist you with monitoring your side effects everyday and recognize their causes.

You can make an objective to compose for a couple of moments every day or week. In particular, what you need to expound on is totally doing you.

14. Take a stab at something new totally

At the point when you do exactly the same thing a large number of days, you utilize similar pieces of your mind. Doing new things can feel fulfilling and may further develop your general prosperity and reinforce your social connections. To receive these rewards, think about attempting another game, innovative class, or cooking procedure.

15. Decide to render help sometimes

You can take out a couple of birds with one stone — investing energy with others and exploring new territory — by chipping in and giving your opportunity to some other person or thing. You might be accustomed to getting help from companions, yet connecting and giving assistance may really further develop your emotional well-being more.

Extra: Individuals who volunteer experience actual advantages as well. This incorporates a brought down chance of hypertension and further developed rest.

16. Practice appreciation

At the point when you accomplish something you love, or in any event, when you find another action you appreciate, you might have the option to help your emotional well-being more by carving out opportunity to be grateful for it.

Rehearsing appreciation can meaningfully affect your by and large emotional wellness.

Additionally, recording your appreciation — remembering for notes to other people — can be especially significant.

17. Integrate contemplation

Stress and tension can draw out your depression side effects. Finding unwinding procedures can assist you with bringing down pressure and welcome more satisfaction and equilibrium into your day.

Research proposes that care exercises might assist you with working on your feeling of prosperity and feel more associated with what's going on around you.

These exercises can include:
- *contemplation*
- *yoga*
- *profound relaxing*
- *journaling*

18. Eat well

There's no enchanted eating routine that will treat discouragement. Be that as it may, what you put into your body can affect the manner in which you feel.

Certain individuals likewise feel improved and have more energy when they keep away from sugar, additives, and handled food sources.

On the off chance that you have the means, think about gathering with a specialist or enlisted dietitian for direction.

Eating an eating regimen wealthy in lean meats, vegetables, and grains might be an extraordinary spot to

begin. Attempt to restrict energizers like caffeine, espresso, and pop and depressants like liquor
Confided in Source

.

19. Think about restricting medications and liquor
Substances, for example, medications or liquor can add to sustaining sensations of trouble.
Then again, individuals who live with dependence might encounter side effects of depression.
You might need to think about restricting or keeping away from the utilization of liquor and different substances to help your burdensome side effects.

20. Practice rest cleanliness
Rest aggravations are normal with discouragement. You may not rest soundly, or you might rest excessively. Both can exacerbate gloom. Go for the gold of rest each evening. Attempt to get into a sound resting schedule.
Hitting the sack and awakening simultaneously consistently can assist you with your everyday timetable. Getting the appropriate measure of rest may likewise assist you with feeling more adjusted and empowered over the course of your day.

22. Consider treatment
You may likewise find it supportive to talk with an expert about the thing you're going through. An overall professional might have the option to allude you to an advisor or other subject matter expert. They can survey your side effects and assist with fostering a clinical treatment plan custom fitted to your necessities. This

might incorporate different choices, like prescription and treatment. Finding the right treatment for you might take some time, so open up to a specialist or medical care proficient about the thing is and isn't working. They'll work with you to track down the most ideal choice.

CHAPTER SEVEN

Prevention and Treatment

There are powerful medicines for discouragement. These incorporate mental treatment and meds. Look for care on the off chance that you have side effects of discouragement.
Mental medicines are the main medicines for discouragement. They can be joined with stimulant meds in moderate and serious sorrow. Upper meds are not required for gentle misery.

Mental medicines can show better approaches for thinking, adapting or connecting with others. They might incorporate talk treatment with experts and managed lay advisors. Talk treatment can occur face to face or on the web. Mental medicines might be gotten to through self improvement manuals, sites and applications.

Among the psychological therapies that work well for depression are:

- stimulation of behavior
- cognitive behavioral treatment
- Problem-solving treatment
- interpersonal psychotherapy.

Antidepressant medications include selective serotonin reuptake inhibitors (SSRIs), such as fluoxetine.
Healthcare providers should keep in mind the possible adverse effects associated with antidepressant medication, the ability to deliver either intervention (in terms of expertise and/or treatment availability), and individual preferences

Antidepressants ought not be utilized for treating depression in youngsters and are not the first line of treatment in quite a while, among whom they ought to be utilized with additional mindfulness.

Various meds and medicines are utilized for bipolar turmoil.

Taking care of oneself
Taking care of oneself can assume a significant part in overseeing side effects of wretchedness and advancing in general prosperity.

What you can do:
- attempt to continue to do exercises you used to appreciate
- stick to standard eating and resting propensities however much as could reasonably be expected

- stay away from or cut down on liquor and don't utilize illegal medications, which can aggravate wretchedness
- converse with somebody you trust about your sentiments
- look for help from a medical services supplier.

On the off chance that you have considerations of self destruction:

- recollect you are in good company, and that many individuals have gone through the thing you're encountering and tracked down help
- converse with somebody you trust about how you feel
- converse with a wellbeing specialist, like a specialist or instructor
- join a care group.
- In the event that you assume you are in impending peril of hurting yourself, contact any suitable crisis administrations or an emergency line.

Further advances

Attempt these methodologies on the off chance that you're feeling discouraged:

Keep in contact

Try not to pull out from life. Mingling can work on your mind-set. Staying in contact with loved ones implies you have somebody to converse with when you feel low.

Be more dynamic

Take up some type of activity. There's proof that exercise can assist with lifting your temperament. In the event that you haven't practiced for some time, begin tenderly by strolling for 20 minutes consistently.

Overcome your apprehensions

Try not to stay away from the things you view as troublesome. At the point when individuals feel low or restless, they some of the time try not to converse with others. Certain individuals can lose their trust in going out, driving or voyaging.

If this begins to occur, looking up to these circumstances will assist them with becoming simpler.

Have a daily practice

At the point when individuals feel down, they can get into unfortunate rest designs, keeping awake until late and dozing during the day. Attempt to get up at your typical time and adhere to your everyday practice however much as could be expected.

Not having a routine can influence your eating. Attempt to continue preparing and eating ordinary dinners.

CHAPTER EIGHT

Conclusion

Depression is a prevalent condition that can lead to suffering, functional impairment, an increased risk of suicide, increased health care expenses, and decreased productivity. There are efficient therapies for both the independent occurrence of depression and its co-occurring general medical conditions. Many cases of depression that are found in normal medical settings can be treated there. In basic care settings, around half of all cases of depression are diagnosed; yet, the therapies that follow frequently do not meet current best practices. Short-term patient outcomes are often satisfactory when treatments with proven efficacy are administered. Stigma, patient somatization and denial, physician knowledge and skill deficiencies, time constraints, lack of providers and treatments, restrictions on third-party coverage, and limitations on specialized, pharmaceutical, and psychotherapeutic care are some of the obstacles to diagnosing and treating depression.

www.ingramcontent.com/pod-product-compliance
Lightning Source LLC
Chambersburg PA
CBHW050758250726

48662CB00005B/2282